THE PARENTS' GUIDE TO

EXPLAINING
SEX

WHAT TO TELL YOUR CHILD AND
5 SIMPLE STEPS TO GET STARTED

CATH HAKANSON

THE PARENTS' GUIDE TO EXPLAINING SEX
by Cath Hakanson

Published by Sex Ed Rescue

PO Box 7903
Cloisters Square WA 6000
Australia

sexedrescue.com

Illustrations by Embla Granqvist
Interior design by Jevgenija Bitter

For permission contact:
cath@sexedrescue.com
ISBN-13: 978-0-6489201-3-7

CONTENTS

INTRODUCTION

Talking to kids about sex is challenging for all parents, regardless of how confident you might think you are. Trust me, I'm a parent myself, and despite being extremely comfortable talking about sex, I sometimes still squirm when my kids ask me certain questions. There was the one from my daughter that left me speechless: 'How many people have you had sex with?' Or, last night, when my 9-year-old son pulled out a book about where babies come from, and I could feel myself getting anxious as we got to the very detailed description of sexual intercourse.

It doesn't matter how comfortable you might think you are; talking about sex with kids just makes you squirm. But luckily, the more you talk about it, the less you squirm!

One of the hardest parts of talking to kids about sex is knowing what exactly to tell them. Will you say the wrong thing? Or give them too much information (or not enough)? Will they actually understand what you are saying?

And once you have decided what to say, **then you need to work out how to start the conversation**!

Which is why I wrote this book – *The Parents' Guide to Explaining Sex.*

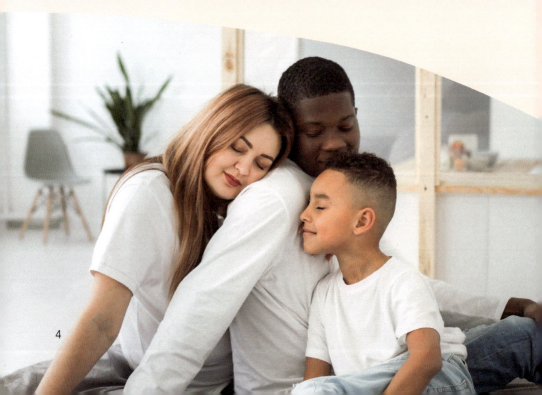

This book will tell you what to tell your child about sex and how to start saying it.

It breaks sexual intercourse into five simple steps so that your child is learning about sex in smaller pieces, where each new piece of information adds to the knowledge they already have. This means that you are giving your child information that they will understand, will make sense and is right for their stage of development. And it doesn't matter how old your child is, as these explanations are suitable for children between the ages of 3 to 12.

There are many ways to explain sex to kids, and this book will provide you with straightforward explanations that are inclusive and based on the latest research, standardised child sexual development milestones, my 25+ years of clinical expertise and the common sense of a parent who does this with her own kids.

The Parents' Guide to Explaining Sex also **helps you to start the conversation** with your child. It provides you with over 20 ways to start talking. Regardless of whether your child is a willing listener or not, these conversation starters will help you to have meaningful conversations with your child.

Let's get started!

Cath

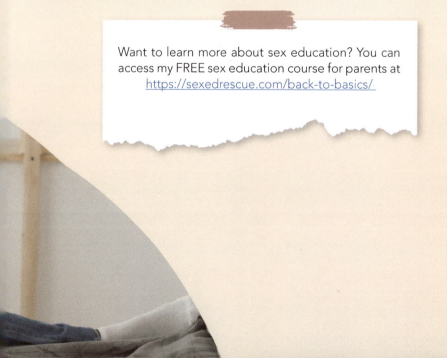

Want to learn more about sex education? You can access my FREE sex education course for parents at
https://sexedrescue.com/back-to-basics/

10 IMPORTANT THINGS TO KNOW BEFORE YOU START

1. **If you don't tell your child about sex, someone else will do it for you.** If your child doesn't hear about sex from their peers at the playground, then they will hear about it on the internet, in music, on advertising and through TV. So, get in first and make sure your child receives the right information about sex.

2. **It is never too late (or too early) to start talking.** It might feel that you have left it too late to start talking, but you haven't. Start talking and let your child know that they can turn to you for support, guidance and information as they grow up. And by talking to kids when they are younger, you're setting yourself up as their trusted source for information and guidance. Which means they're less likely to seek out other inaccurate and misleading sources of information from their peers, media, and the Internet if they think of you as their "go-to" person.

3. **It is an everyday conversation.** Today, it is about many conversations (not just one talk) about sex that happen until your child leaves home. Which means that it doesn't matter if you forget to say something (or stuff it up), as there will be many more opportunities to talk again. Talk in the same tone and with the same language that you normally use.

4. **Be prepared to repeat these conversations.** Kids will either sift through all the information or let it pass. They may come back to you later on for more information about something that they are still curious about.

5. **Information about sex is helpful (not harmful) to children.** One of the biggest fears parents have about sex education is that they are giving their child permission to be sexual. Or even worse, that they are suggesting that they be sexual. Research[1] tells us that children whose parents speak openly about sex with them will postpone involvement in sexual activities until they are older, and act with more responsibility if and when they become involved.

1. https://sexedrescue.com/advantages-of-sex-education/

6. **Sharing of values provides your child with a moral compass.** Share what sexual attitudes and behaviours are okay (and not okay) in your family, and why. You'll be providing them with a moral compass to guide them as they make sense of the mixed messages that they will receive from the media, their peers, and the world around them.

7. **Use simple and age-appropriate language.** Keep your words simple and factual, i.e., no storks, cabbage patches or special cuddles, as that just confuses them. Don't try to cover everything at once, but also don't worry if you think you have said too much (as kids quickly forget anything that is more than they can understand).

8. **Don't wait for your child to ask the first question.** Some kids will ask, but some kids won't. By waiting, you're practically guaranteeing that their first sources of knowledge will not be you. Many kids are predictable and will start asking a series of questions from the age of 3-6 about where babies come from. So, take advantage of it and let their questions guide the conversation.

9. **You're teaching your child about the creation of life (not how to have sex).** Talking to kids about 'where they came from' is very different than 'adult sex'. To kids, it's about the science of how new life is created. As they grow up, you'll be able to help them understand that there is more to sex than making babies.

10. **It's the conversation that matters (not the facts you share).** Don't get caught up in the details of what to say and how to say it. What matters is the fact that you're talking about a topic that is seen as taboo. You might feel as if you are fumbling along, or that you could have explained things a bit better, but your child won't see that. They'll see you as 'askable,' which means that they'll know that if you can talk about sex, that they can talk to you about anything (no matter what).

HOW TO EXPLAIN SEX TO KIDS

When explaining sex to kids, we don't have to go straight into a detailed description of sexual intercourse. Instead, we start off with the basics, and if your child wants to know more, you then provide them with more information, gradually filling in the gaps until they understand it.

WHY DO WE BREAK SEX INTO A SERIES OF STEPS?

There are a few reasons why I like to break sex into a series of steps.

Firstly, because it makes it a lot easier for you, the parent! Most parents struggle with talking to their kids about sex for many different reasons[1]. The biggest hurdle for parents, though, is the fear that they will be sexualising their child by giving them too much information about sex. By breaking sex down into simple information, it means that we can start off by talking about the easier (and less threatening) parts before you get into a fully detailed description.

Secondly, the easiest way to get comfortable with talking to kids about sex is to slowly desensitize yourself. Desensitization is defined as the diminished emotional responsiveness to a negative, aversive or positive stimulus after repeated exposure to it[2]. This means that the more you talk about sex with your kids, the easier it gets. I find that by breaking sex down into simple steps, it gives you time to get comfortable with the easier stuff, so that by the time you get to the trickier stuff, you'll find talking much easier.

Thirdly, kids learn differently from how adults learn. True understanding is a gradual process of learning[3]. This means that we don't give them all the information at once, as their degree of understanding is much simpler and more concrete than ours. We start off with basic facts that we keep on repeating, gradually adding in more information as we see them understanding what we have to say. As your child's parent, you're the best judge of what they do and don't understand. Trust your gut instinct and remember that even if you do give them too much information, you won't be harming them. We are all guilty of sometimes giving too much information, and your child will just forget what you have said, as it won't make much sense at all. We all learn from our mistakes, and parenting is full of them!

1. https://sexedrescue.com/myths-and-facts-about-sex/
2. https://en.wikipedia.org/wiki/Desensitization_(psychology)
3. https://www.heysigmund.com/developmental-stage/

WHAT IF MY CHILD ISN'T READY TO HEAR ABOUT SEX?

You can't give kids too much information about sex. Just like other subjects, if kids hear information from a calm, caring adult that is beyond their ability to absorb or understand, they'll simply become bored and turn their attention elsewhere. So, try to keep it age-appropriate, but don't stress if you do give too much information, as it happens all the time!

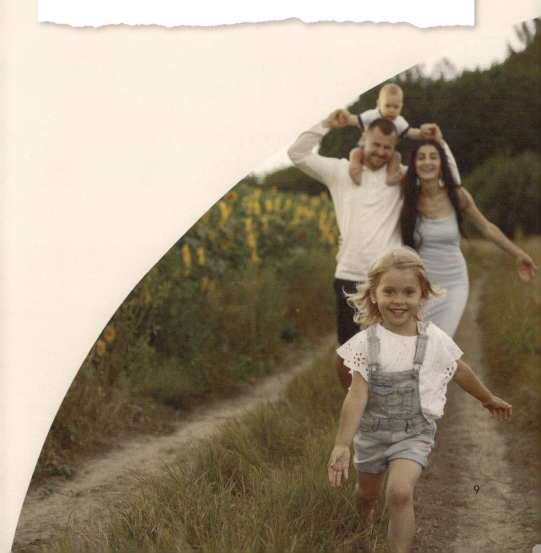

5 STEPS TO EXPLAINING SEXUAL INTERCOURSE

You will find two sets of explanations. The **'Common Explanations'** (which uses the language that many of us are familiar with) and the **'Inclusive Explanations'** (which uses language that is inclusive for trans gender and nonbinary people).

When we first start talking about sex with kids, we talk about baby-making sex. Why? Because it is developmentally appropriate for young children to be curious about where babies come from. And sex is an easier concept for them to understand (and for us to explain) when we explain it as baby-making. As they get older, we then add in that sex is much more than just penises and vaginas, and that adults have sex for reasons other than making babies.

But isn't there more to sex than making babies?

Yes, there is a lot more to sex than making babies. And once your child understands what sex is, you can then add in this extra information.

STEP 1: WHERE BABIES COME FROM.

Initially, a child's curiosity is aroused because they are trying to work out where they were before they were born. The first thing they usually want to know is, **where do babies come from?**

STEP 2: WHAT MAKES A BABY.

But then, they start to think about it a little bit more. So, they understand that they grew inside a uterus, but they want to know what made them grow, i.e., how did they happen or start? They want to know, **what makes a baby?**

STEP 3: WHERE THE SPERM & EGG COME FROM.

Next, they might start to wonder **where the sperm & egg come from.**

STEP 4: HOW THE SPERM & EGG MEET.

Eventually, they'll want to know **how the sperm & egg meet!** How does the sperm get from the testicles to the egg in the fallopian tubes?

STEP 5: WHAT SEX IS.

Then, they want to try and understand the mechanics of how a baby is made through **sexual intercourse**. With this last step, it might feel that this is when we get into a fully detailed explanation of sexual intercourse. Well, you can relax, because you don't have to just yet, as we can talk to kids about it gradually. We can start with a basic explanation, and if your child wants to know more, you then provide them with more information, gradually filling in the gaps until they understand it.

Don't expect your child to understand sex immediately. Sexual intercourse is a difficult concept for kids to understand. They see it as some weird (or totally gross) thing that adults do. They don't understand why we would want to do it (other than to make babies) or how it can make us feel. Their brain isn't wired to think about sex until puberty, which is when sex will start to make a lot more sense to them. Most kids don't understand sex properly until their mid-teens.

Remember that every child is different. Some will have lots of questions, and some won't. And some children will be more curious about sexuality than others – all is normal! You are the best judge of your child's level of development and understanding. So, when looking at what information to give your child, start at the point that feels comfortable.

When looking at the explanations of sex, it is important to remember that each child develops at their own pace. So, your child may (or may not) be ready for some information. Start with the information that feels appropriate for you and your child. At the end of the day, you know your child best!

BEING INCLUSIVE:
A DIFFERENT WAY TO TALK ABOUT SEX

Not a lot has changed with sex over the years. It is still the same body parts doing the same things.

But the way we talk about sex has changed dramatically! Especially regarding the use of gendered language, e.g., mother, father, boys, girls, women, men.

As parents, many of us grew up being taught that girls have vulvas and boys have penises. And that women become pregnant and give birth to babies. And back then, that was true.

But today, that is no longer true.

We now have trans-men and non-binary people becoming pregnant, birthing and direct-feeding their own babies. We also see trans-women direct feeding babies with the help of medication. Today, we are talking in a more inclusive way.

A trans-man is a person born with a vulva (and assigned the sex of female at birth) but who identifies as a man (not a woman).

A trans-woman is a person with a penis (and assigned the sex of male at birth) but who identifies as a woman (not a man).

A non-binary person is someone who doesn't identify exclusively as a man or a woman. They might feel like a mix of genders or like they have no gender at all.

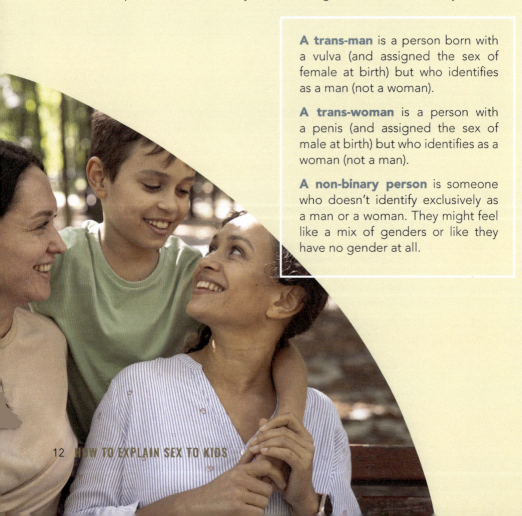

By inclusive, I mean by talking in a way that includes everyone (and doesn't exclude anyone). For example, when I talk about women being pregnant, that excludes non-binary and transgender people. When I talk about people with a uterus being pregnant, that includes everyone.

SO HOW DO I ANSWER QUESTIONS LIKE, "CAN A MAN BE PREGNANT?"

The way we used to answer this question would be, "No, men can't grow a baby". But technically this is inaccurate, as some men with a uterus can be pregnant. And it isn't inclusive of all people.

An accurate way to answer this question could be, "No, most men can't grow a baby. You need a uterus to grow a baby."

An inclusive way to answer this question could be, "You need a uterus to grow a baby. So, if a man has a uterus, then he could grow a baby."

BUT WON'T I CONFUSE MY CHILD?

A lot of parents worry that kids will get confused about this. I have found that often it is the parents who are confused, and not the kids! If kids can understand that not all kids have a mummy and a daddy, and that some have one mummy, and some may have two daddies, then they can understand that it takes a uterus to grow a baby and that gender has nothing to do with it!

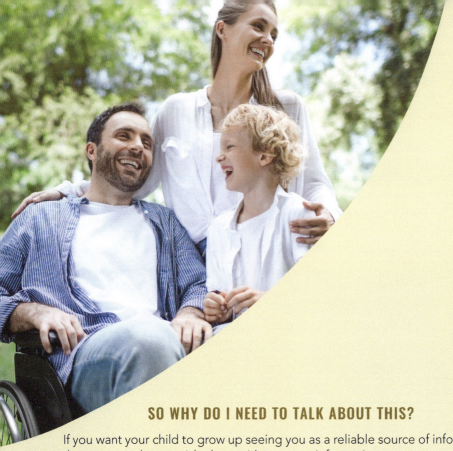

SO WHY DO I NEED TO TALK ABOUT THIS?

If you want your child to grow up seeing you as a reliable source of information, then you need to provide them with accurate information.

You may think that this conversation is irrelevant as you may not personally know a transgender or non-binary person. But as your child has more exposure to the outside world, it is possible that they may see a pregnant man on the news or at your local shops. Or they may have a family member disclose that they are transgender or non-binary.

You may believe that only women can be pregnant, and not men. Regardless of what you believe, this is something that exists, i.e., it is a fact. And this fact does not stop you from sharing your values and beliefs.

I am a firm believer that parents need to provide kids with factual information. If you want your child to see you as a reliable source of information and to turn to you with their questions (instead of their friends or the internet), then you need to answer their questions honestly and provide them with accurate facts.

Plus, if you want your child to grow up into an adult who treats people fairly and doesn't discriminate based on their gender or sex, then it is important to talk in an inclusive way. With the focus on anti-bullying and diversity and inclusion in schools and workplaces, it's important that children learn how to understand and interact with people of all backgrounds.

PLEASE READ THIS
IF YOU ARE FEELING OVERWHELMED

Explaining sex can be very overwhelming. And the thought of explaining it in an inclusive way may make it feel impossible to get started.

So rather than put the sex conversation into the 'too hard' basket, I'd like to suggest that you take it one step at a time.

Your priority is to start explaining sex. So, start off with the 'Common Explanations' (which use the language that many of us are familiar with).

Once you've had a few conversations and you begin to feel more comfortable with talking to your child about sex, you can start talking in a more inclusive way by referring to the 'Inclusive Explanations'.

At first it may feel a little clumsy saying 'person with a uterus' instead of woman, but over time, you will get more used to it.

And in case you're wondering whether your child will get confused (or not) by a change in information, they usually don't. They are already used to us changing things on them regarding other things, such as what they can and can't eat, what movies they can and can't watch, where they can and can't ride their bikes, etc.

A lot of parents worry that their child will be confused by a change in language and facts. They usually aren't, and if they do get confused, then a few corrections are all that's needed to explain.

COMMON EXPLANATIONS

Uses language that many of us are familiar with

STEP 1.
WHERE BABIES COME FROM

Let your child know what is socially acceptable. For example, some adults don't like to hear kids using words like penis in the playground. Or, that some parents like to talk to their own kids about how babies are made.

There is more than one way to explain where babies come from. So, use the explanation that you feel most comfortable with.

Babies come from inside the mommy.

Babies come from inside the mommy, near the belly.

Babies come from a special place inside the mommy.

The place where babies grow is called the uterus (or womb).

The uterus is the place where babies grow.

ANOTHER WORD FOR UTERUS IS WOMB.

Grab a balloon and blow it up whilst explaining to your child that the uterus is like a balloon; it stretches as the baby grows bigger and bigger.

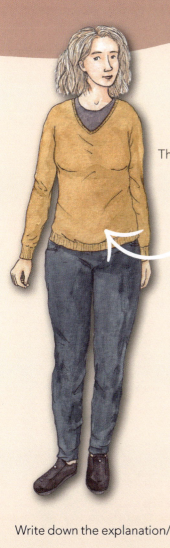

The uterus lives here.

This is what a uterus looks like if you could see inside the body.

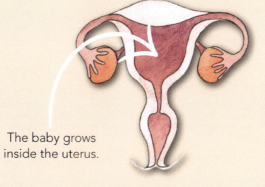

The baby grows inside the uterus.

Write down the explanation/s you would like to use:

_____

_____

_____

_____

_____

WHAT MAKES A BABY

There is more than one way to explain what makes a baby. So, use the explanation that you feel most comfortable with.

You'll find some examples of different language to use with your child. Start with the words that you are ready to use. Then, as you become more comfortable with those words, start to use the next set of words.

2 PEOPLE

You can also say 'a man and a woman' or 'a mommy and a daddy', but it is important to remember that not all babies are made this way. Some families might have two mommies, or two daddies, or just one mommy or one daddy. So just use the language that suits your family.

You need a man and a woman to make a baby. Together, they can make a baby.

You need a grown-up man and a grown-up woman to make a baby.

Remind your child that making babies is something that only adults do. Get into the habit of saying, 'Only adults can make babies (not kids).'

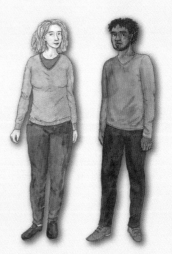

PARTS

It takes two parts to make a baby. A part from a man and a part from a woman.

CELLS

A baby starts off as a tiny cell. Half of this cell comes from the woman and the other half comes from the man. They join, then together, they grow into a baby.

SPERM & EGG (OVUM)

The proper name for the egg is ovum, but everyone calls it an egg. Sometimes you will hear sperm referred to as a seed.

You need a sperm and an egg to make a baby.

You need a sperm from a man and an egg from a woman to make a baby.

A sperm from the man needs to join with an egg from the woman to make a baby.

When the sperm and egg join together, a baby starts to form.

The sperm and the egg are both tiny.

3 THINGS

You need three things to make a baby. Sperm, an egg, and a place for the baby to grow (the uterus).

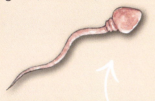

1. This is a sperm cell.

2. This is an egg cell.

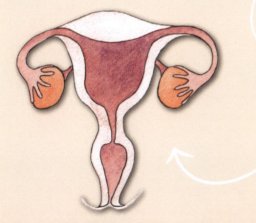

3. This is what the uterus looks like inside the body.

Write down the explanation/s you would like to use:

_____

_____

_____

_____

_____

WHERE THE SPERM AND EGG COME FROM

There is more than one way to explain where the sperm and egg come from. So, use the explanation that you feel most comfortable with.

This time, we are just telling them where the parts that make a baby come from. Some kids will be happy with just this, but others will also want to know how the two parts meet.

SPERM

The sperm come from a man.

The sperm are made in the testicles and come out through the penis.

There are two testicles and they are found in the scrotum.

If your child has testicles, ask them if they can feel them through their scrotum. It will feel like a boiled egg that has been peeled (but much smaller) or like a grape. Soft but firm and a little squishy.

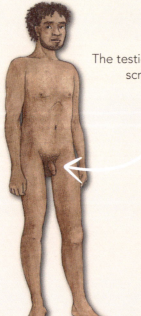

The testicles sit inside the scrotum here.

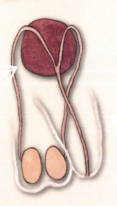

Bladder

Penis

Testicles

EGG

The egg comes from a woman.

The eggs are stored inside the ovaries.

There are two ovaries.

The ovaries are inside the body here.

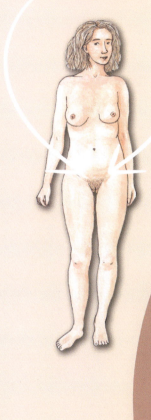

Fallopian Tube

Uterus

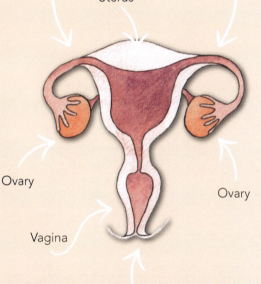

Ovary

Ovary

Vagina

Vulva

Write down the explanation/s you would like to use:

_____

_____

_____

_____

_____

STEP 4.
HOW THE SPERM AND EGG MEET

There is more than one way to explain how the sperm and egg meet. So, use the explanation that you feel comfortable with using.

Babies can be made in lots of different ways: natural conception, sperm and/or egg donation, assisted reproductive technology, surrogacy, adoption.

You'll find some examples of different language to use with your child. Start with the words that you are ready to use. Then, as you become more comfortable with those words, start to use the next set of words.

PENIS IN VAGINA

There are two ways to talk about sexual intercourse. We can talk about the penis being placed in the vagina. Or we can talk about the woman letting the man place his penis into her vagina. The second explanation informs a child that sex is consensual and something that both people agree to.

You can name this behaviour if you want to, e.g. 'This is called sex'. They may ask for more information, or they may not. So be prepared, just in case!

SPERM

The man puts his sperm inside the woman.

The woman lets the man put his sperm inside her (or inside her vagina).

The woman helps the man to put his sperm inside her.

The woman helps the man to put his sperm inside her vagina.

PENIS

The man puts his penis inside the woman.

The woman lets the man put his penis in her vagina.

The woman helps the man to put his penis inside her vagina.

WHAT HAPPENS NEXT?

Once the sperm are inside the woman, they travel inside her towards the egg.

A baby is made when sperm from the penis joins with the egg, which is inside the woman.

The sperm come from the penis. Sperm are in the semen that comes out of the end of a penis.

The sperm travel from the testicles through the penis, then into the vagina. They use their wriggly tails to swim inside, where they meet the egg.

OTHER WAYS TO MAKE A BABY

If your child was made a different way, you can also explain to them how they were made.

Sometimes, the sperm or egg might not work properly, or a person might not have an egg or sperm of their own. Alternatively, a person might be unable to grow a baby inside their body.

To get around these problems, someone might give them an egg or sperm or offer to grow a baby inside their own uterus for them.

A doctor can help by placing the sperm inside the uterus. They may need to help the sperm and egg to join together (this can happen inside or outside the body).

They might need to use special equipment to help people make a baby.

Some people might need special medicine to help them make a baby.

SPERM AND/OR EGG DONATION

Babies can be made in lots of different ways, but we needed some help to make you. Someone gave us some sperm/eggs, and some doctors helped us to make you.

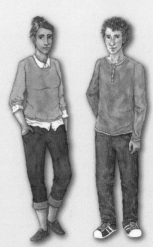

ASSISTED REPRODUCTIVE TECHNOLOGY

Babies can be made in lots of different ways, but we needed some help to make you. A doctor helped to get the sperm and egg to meet, and then they put you in my uterus, which is where you grew.

SURROGACY

Babies can be made in lots of different ways, but we needed some help to make you. We didn't have a uterus, so we found a nice woman who grew you inside her until you were born. A doctor helped to get the sperm and egg to meet, and then put you inside the nice woman's uterus, which is where you grew.

ADOPTION

The sperm and egg that made you didn't come from us. You were already growing in the uterus of the woman who gave birth to you.

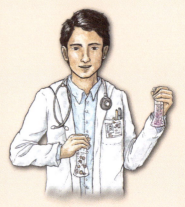

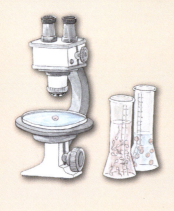

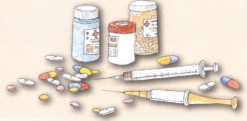

You can find children's books that will help with explaining the way your child was made at http://booksfordonoroffspring. blogspot.com.au/

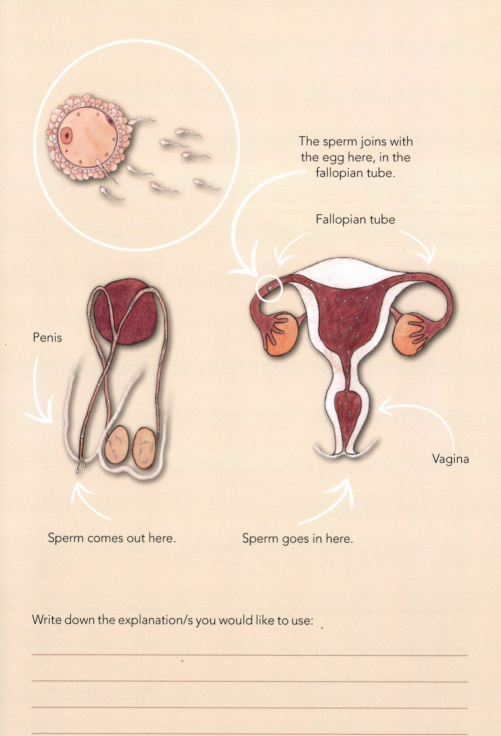

The sperm joins with the egg here, in the fallopian tube.

Fallopian tube

Penis

Vagina

Sperm comes out here.

Sperm goes in here.

Write down the explanation/s you would like to use:

_____

_____

_____

_____

_____

STEP 5.
WHAT SEX IS

There is more than one way to explain sexual intercourse. So, use the explanation that you feel most comfortable with.

The easiest way to talk about sex is by explaining it as a way to make a baby, with a penis going into a vagina. Why? Because it then gives sex a purpose that children can easily understand. Once they understand that concept, we can then start to include that there is a bit more to sex, like hugging & kissing, that two people of the same sex can have sex together, and that adults also have sex for other reasons as well. And don't forget to remind your child that sex is something that adults do, and that it is not for kids.

A 'VAGUE' DESCRIPTION

Sexual intercourse is a way that a man and a woman can make a baby.

Sexual intercourse is something that adults can do when they want to make a baby.

A WAY TO MAKE A BABY

A man and a woman can make a baby by having sex. The penis is placed inside the vagina. The sperm then travel from the testicles through the penis, then into the vagina. The sperm swim into the uterus and fallopian tubes, where they might meet an egg.

A man and a woman can make a baby by having sex. They will kiss and cuddle until the penis become hard and pokes out. Then they put the penis inside the vagina. The sperm will travel from the testicles and out through the penis, then into the vagina. The sperm will use their wriggly tails to swim inside, where they meet the egg.

SOMETHING THAT ADULTS ENJOY

Sex or sexual intercourse is something that adults do to show that they love each other. They will hug, kiss and touch each other's bodies until the penis becomes stiff and the vagina becomes wet and slippery. They will hold each other close and the woman will help to push the penis inside their vagina. They will move their bodies together so that the penis slides in and out of the vagina in a way that feels nice. Eventually sperm will travel from the testicles and out through the penis, and into the vagina.

Sex or sexual intercourse is something that adults do when they want to make a baby or show that they care for each other. They usually find somewhere private, like their bedroom, and will take their clothes off. They will hug and kiss and touch each other's bodies all over until the penis is erect and the vagina is wet and slippery. They will lie close to each other and the woman will help the man to push his penis into her vagina. They will then move their bodies together until the man ejaculates.

What's ejaculate? Or ejaculation? It is when semen, which contains sperm, come out of the penis really fast. There is usually a good feeling that goes with it called an orgasm.

AN EXPLANATION THAT INCLUDES ORGASM

When two adults like each other a lot, they may want to have sexual intercourse with each other. This means that they may hug, kiss and touch each other's bodies all over. The penis becomes erect, and the vagina becomes moist and slippery. This makes it easier for the penis to go into the vagina. The man pushes his penis into the vagina, they hold each other close, they move around a bit, and it can feel good. After a while, the man almost always ejaculates.

Sex usually starts off when the man and woman kiss, hug and touch each other's bodies. They will take their clothes off. This can be a really nice feeling that helps the penis to become stiff and the vagina to become wet and slippery. They will lie close to each other and the woman will help the man to push his penis into her vagina. They will then move their bodies together, with the penis pushing up and down inside the vagina. This gives them both a very nice tingly, excited feeling. As the feeling gets stronger and stronger, they both move faster and faster until the sperm suddenly leaves the testicles and comes out of the penis really fast into the vagina.

What's an erection? An erection is when the penis becomes stiff and pokes out.

SEX BETWEEN 2 PEOPLE OF THE SAME SEX

Sex is something that happens between two people. Those two people might be a man and a woman, two men or two women.

Sex is a way to make a baby but it is also something that two people do to share their love with each other. They will hug, kiss and touch each other's bodies in a way that feels nice. They might kiss the other person's penis, vulva and/or anus. They might place something like their fingers or a penis into the mouth, vagina, and/or anus.

Sex between two men will start when they kiss, hug and touch each other's bodies. They will take their clothes off and they may touch each other's penis with their hands and mouth. Sometimes they might push their erect penis into the other person's bottom. They may touch each other's penises in a way that feels so nice that the sperm will rush through the testicles and out of the penis really fast.

Sex between two women will start when they kiss, hug and touch each other's bodies. They will take their clothes off and they may touch each other's vulvas with their hands and mouth. Sometimes they might push their fingers into the other person's vagina. They may touch each other's vulvas in a way that gives them a nice tingly feeling all over their body.

- Sex is only for adults, not children.
- Sex is something that adults do because they like it.
- Sex is a private activity that people do when they are alone.
- A baby is not made every time people have sex.
- Adults can stop a baby from being made by using contraception (special medicine or ways to prevent pregnancy).

Some kids will get stressed about sex. They will worry about having to do it. They forget that by the time they are ready to be sexual with a partner, that they will have an adult body, an adult brain and feelings that are ready for sex. They also need to be reminded that they don't have to have sex if they don't want to.

Write down the explanation/s you would like to use:

_____

_____

_____

_____

_____

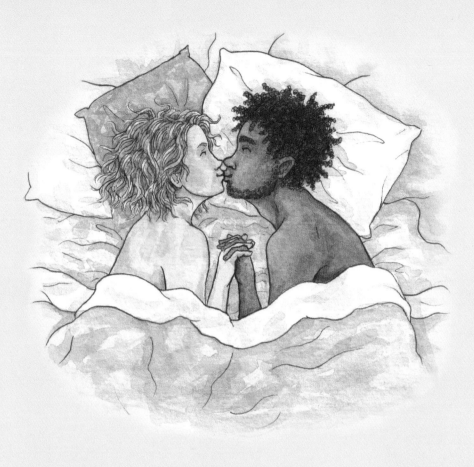

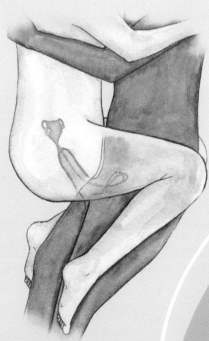

INCLUSIVE EXPLANATIONS

Uses language that is inclusive for trans gender and nonbinary people

WHERE BABIES COME FROM

Let your child know what is socially acceptable. For example, some adults don't like to hear kids using words like penis in the playground. Or, that some parents like to talk to their own kids about how babies are made.

There is more than one way to explain where babies come from. So, use the explanation that you feel most comfortable with.

Babies come from inside the body of a person with a uterus.

Babies come from inside the uterus, which is near the belly.

Babies come from a special place called the uterus.

The place where babies grow is called the uterus (or womb).

The uterus is the place where babies grow.

ANOTHER WORD FOR UTERUS IS WOMB.

Grab a balloon and blow it up whilst explaining to your child that the uterus is like a balloon; it stretches as the baby grows bigger and bigger.

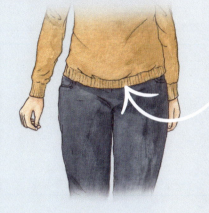

The uterus lives here.

This is what a uterus looks like if you could see inside the body.

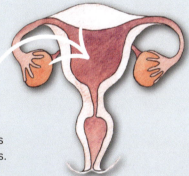

The baby grows inside the uterus.

Write down the explanation/s you would like to use:

_____

_____

_____

_____

_____

STEP 2.
WHAT MAKES A BABY

There is more than one way to explain what makes a baby. So, use the explanation that you feel most comfortable with.

You'll find some examples of different language to use with your child. Start with the words that you are ready to use. Then, as you become more comfortable with those words, start to use the next set of words.

2 PEOPLE

There are many different ways to describe the people with the necessary parts to make a baby.

For the person providing the eggs, you can say a person with ovaries, or a uterus, or a vulva, or a vagina.

For the person providing the sperm, you can say a person with testicles or a penis.

Remind your child that making babies is something that only adults do. Get into the habit of always saying, 'Only adults can make babies (not kids).'

What words will you use to describe a person with eggs? A person with

What words will you use to describe a person with sperms? A person with

It is also important to remember that not all babies are made with two people. One person can decide to make a baby by using someone else's sperm, eggs and/or uterus. So, use the language that suits your family.

You need two people to make a baby. One person has to have ovaries while the other person has to have testicles.

You need a person with testicles and a person with a uterus to make a baby. Together, they can make a baby.

You need a grown-up person with a penis and a grown-up person with a vulva to make a baby.

PARTS

It takes two parts to make a baby. A part from a person with testicles and another part from a person with ovaries.

CELLS

A baby starts off as a tiny cell. Half of this cell comes from a person with a uterus and the other half comes from a person with testicles. The two parts join, then together, they grow into a baby.

SPERM & EGG (OVUM)

The proper name for the egg is ovum, but everyone calls it an egg. Sometimes you will hear sperm referred to as a seed.

You need a sperm and an egg to make a baby.

You need a sperm from the testicles and an egg from the ovaries to make a baby.

A sperm needs to join with an egg to make a baby.

A sperm from the testicles needs to join with an egg from the ovaries to make a baby.

When the sperm and egg join together, a baby starts to form.

The sperm and the egg are both tiny.

3 THINGS

You need three things to make a baby. Sperm, an egg and a place for the baby to grow (the uterus).

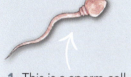

1. This is a sperm cell.

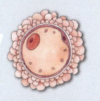

2. This is an egg cell.

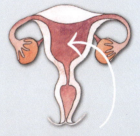

3. This is what the uterus looks like inside the body.

Write down the explanation/s you would like to use:

_____

_____

_____

_____

_____

STEP 3.
WHERE THE SPERM AND EGG COME FROM

There is more than one way to explain where the sperm and egg come from. So, use the explanation that you feel most comfortable with.

This time, we are just telling them where the parts that make a baby come from. Some kids will be happy with just this, but others will also want to know how the two parts meet.

SPERM

The sperm come from a person with testicles.

The sperm are made in the testicles and come out through the penis.

There are two testicles and they are found in the scrotum.

If your child has testicles, ask them if they can feel them through their scrotum. It will feel like a boiled egg that has been peeled (but much smaller) or like a grape. Soft but firm and a little squishy.

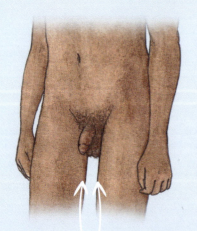

The testicles sit inside the scrotum here.

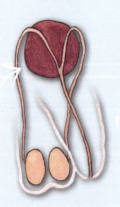

Bladder

Penis

Testicles

EGG

The egg comes from a person with ovaries.

The eggs are stored inside the ovaries.

There are two ovaries.

The ovaries are inside the body here.

Fallopian Tube

Uterus

Ovary

Ovary

Vagina

Vulva

Write down the explanation/s you would like to use:

_____

_____

_____

_____

_____

STEP 4.
HOW THE SPERM AND EGG MEET

There is more than one way to explain how the sperm and egg meet. So, use the explanation that you feel comfortable with using.

Babies can be made in lots of different ways: natural conception, sperm and/or egg donation, assisted reproductive technology, surrogacy, adoption.

You'll find some examples of different language to use with your child. Start with the words that you are ready to use. Then, as you become more comfortable with those words, start to use the next set of words.

PENIS IN VAGINA

There are two ways to talk about sexual intercourse. We can talk about the penis being placed in the vagina. Or we can talk about someone allowing the other person to place their penis into their vagina. The second explanation informs a child that sex is consensual and something that both people agree to.

You can name this behaviour if you want to, e.g. 'This is called sex'. They may ask for more information, or they may not. So be prepared, just in case!

SPERM

The person with the sperm places it inside the other person.

The person with the egg lets the other person place their sperm inside them (or inside their vagina).

The person with the egg helps the other person to put their sperm inside them.

The person with the egg helps the other person to put their sperm inside their vagina.

PENIS

The person with the sperm places their penis inside the other person.

The person with the egg lets the other person place their penis in their vagina.

The person with the egg helps the other person to put their penis inside their vagina.

WHAT HAPPENS NEXT?

Once the sperm is inside the vagina, they travel inside them towards the egg.

A baby is made when sperm from the penis joins with the egg, which is inside the person with the uterus.

The sperm come from the testicles. Sperm are in the semen that comes out of the end of a penis.

The sperm travel from the testicles through the penis, then into the vagina. They use their wriggly tails to swim inside, where they meet the egg.

OTHER WAYS TO MAKE A BABY

If your child was made a different way, you can also explain to them how they were made.

Sometimes, the sperm or egg might not work properly, or a person might not have an egg or sperm of their own. Alternatively, a person might be unable to grow a baby inside their body.

To get around these problems, someone might give them an egg or a sperm, or offer to grow a baby inside their own uterus for them.

A doctor can help by placing the sperm inside the uterus. They may need to help the sperm and egg to join together (this can happen inside or outside the body).

They might need to use special equipment to help someone make a baby.

Some people might need special medicine to help them make a baby.

SPERM AND/OR EGG DONATION

Babies can be made in lots of different ways, but we needed some help to make you. Someone gave us some sperm/eggs, and some doctors helped us to make you.

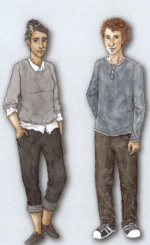

ASSISTED REPRODUCTIVE TECHNOLOGY

Babies can be made in lots of different ways, but we needed some help to make you. A doctor helped to get the sperm and egg to meet, and then they put you in my uterus, which is where you grew.

SURROGACY

Babies can be made in lots of different ways, but we needed some help to make you. We didn't have a uterus, so we found a nice person who grew you inside their uterus until you were born. A doctor helped to get the sperm and egg to meet, and then put you inside the nice person's uterus, which is where you grew.

ADOPTION

The sperm and egg that made you didn't come from us. You were already growing in the uterus of the person who gave birth to you.

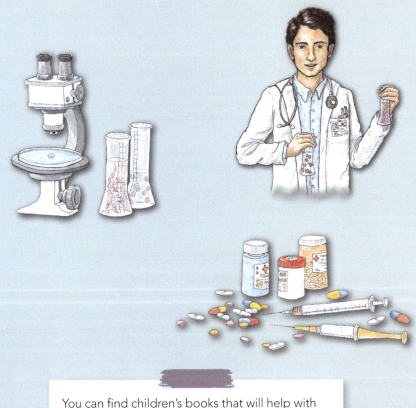

You can find children's books that will help with explaining the way your child was made at http://booksfordonoroffspring.blogspot.com.au/

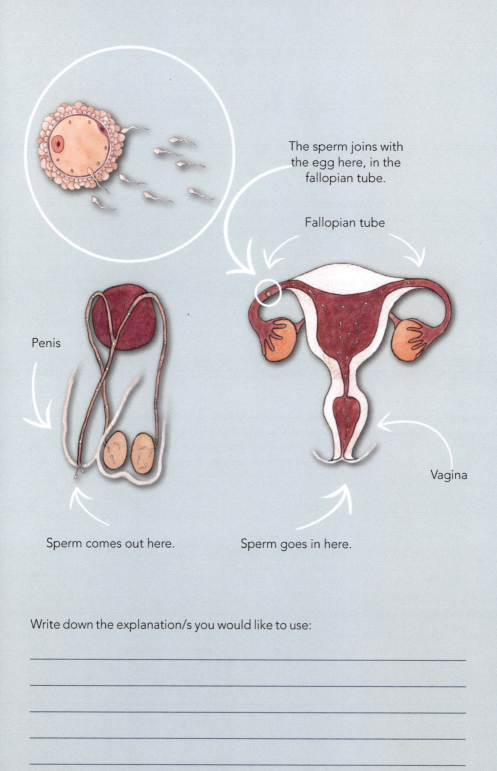

The sperm joins with the egg here, in the fallopian tube.

Fallopian tube

Penis

Vagina

Sperm comes out here.

Sperm goes in here.

Write down the explanation/s you would like to use:

_____

_____

_____

_____

_____

WHAT SEX IS

There is more than one way to explain sexual intercourse. So, use the explanation that you feel most comfortable with.

The easiest way to talk about sex is by explaining it as a way to make a baby, with a penis going into a vagina. Why? Because it then gives sex a purpose that children can easily understand. Once they understand that concept, we can then start to include that there is a bit more to sex, like hugging & kissing, that two people of the same sex can have sex together, and that adults also have sex for other reasons as well. And don't forget to remind your child that sex is something that adults do, and that it is not for kids.

A 'VAGUE' DESCRIPTION

Sexual intercourse is a way that two people can make a baby.

Sexual intercourse is something that adults can do when they want to make a baby.

A WAY TO MAKE A BABY

Two people can make a baby by having sex. The penis is placed inside the vagina. The sperm then travel from the testicles through the penis and into the vagina. The sperm swim into the uterus and fallopian tubes, where they might meet an egg.

A person with a penis and a person with a vagina can make a baby by having sex. They will kiss and cuddle until the penis become hard and pokes out. Then they put the penis inside the vagina. The sperm will travel from the testicles and out through the penis, and into the vagina. The sperm will use their wriggly tails to swim inside, where they meet the egg.

SOMETHING THAT ADULTS ENJOY

Sex or sexual intercourse is something that adults do to show that they love each other. They will hug, kiss and touch each other's bodies until the penis becomes stiff and the vagina becomes wet and slippery. They will hold each other close and the person with the vagina will help to push the penis inside their vagina. They will move their bodies together so that the penis slides in and out of the vagina in a way that feels nice. Eventually sperm will travel from the testicles, out through the penis, and into the vagina.

Sex or sexual intercourse is something that adults do when they want to make a baby or show that they care for each other. They usually find somewhere private, like their bedroom, and will take their clothes off. They will hug and kiss and touch each other's bodies all over until the penis is erect and the vagina is wet and slippery. They will lie close to each other and together they will push the penis into the vagina. They will then move their bodies together until the man ejaculates.

What's ejaculate? Or ejaculation? It is when semen, which contains sperm, come out of the penis really fast. There is usually a good feeling that goes with it called an orgasm.

AN EXPLANATION THAT INCLUDES ORGASM

When two adults like each other a lot, they may want to have sexual intercourse with each other. This means that they may hug, kiss and touch each other's bodies all over. The penis becomes erect, and the vagina becomes moist and slippery. This makes it easier for the penis to go into the vagina. They will push the penis into the vagina, they hold each other close, they move around a bit, and it can feel good. After a while, the person with the penis almost always ejaculates.

Sex usually starts off when the two people kiss, hug and touch each other's bodies. They will take their clothes off. This can be a really nice feeling that helps the penis to become stiff and the vagina to become wet and slippery. They will lie close to each other and the person with the vagina will help the other person to push their penis into the

What's an erection? An erection is when the penis becomes stiff and pokes out.

vagina. They will then move their bodies together, with the penis pushing up and down inside the vagina. This gives them both a very nice tingly, excited feeling. As the feeling gets stronger and stronger, they both move faster and faster until the sperm suddenly leaves the testicles and comes out of the penis really fast into the vagina.

SEX BETWEEN 2 PEOPLE OF THE SAME SEX

Sex is something that happens between two people. Those two people might be a person with a penis and a person with a vagina, two people with penises or two people with vaginas.

Sex is a way to make a baby but it is also something that two people do to share their love with each other. They will hug, kiss and touch each other's bodies in a way that feels nice. They might kiss the other person's penis, vulva and/or anus. They might place something like their fingers or a penis into the mouth, vagina, and/or anus.

Sex between two people with penises will start when they kiss, hug and touch each other's bodies. They will take their clothes off and they may touch each other's penis with their hands and mouth. Sometimes, they might push their erect penis into the other person's bottom. They may touch each other's penises in a way that feels so nice that the sperm will rush through the testicles and out of the penis really fast.

Sex between two people with vaginas will start when they kiss, hug and touch each other's bodies. They will take their clothes off and they may touch each other's vulvas with their hands and mouth. Sometimes they might push their fingers into the other person's vagina. They may touch each other's vulvas in a way that gives them a nice tingly feeling all over their body.

- Sex is only for adults, not children.
- Sex is something that adults do because they like it.
- Sex is a private activity that people do when they are alone.
- A baby is not made every time people have sex.
- Adults can stop a baby from being made by using contraception (special medicine or ways to prevent pregnancy).

Some kids will get stressed about sex. They will worry about having to do it. They forget that by the time they are ready to be sexual with a partner, that they will have an adult body, an adult brain and feelings that are ready for sex. They also need to be reminded that they don't have to have sex if they don't want to.

Write down the explanation/s you would like to use:

_____

_____

_____

_____

_____

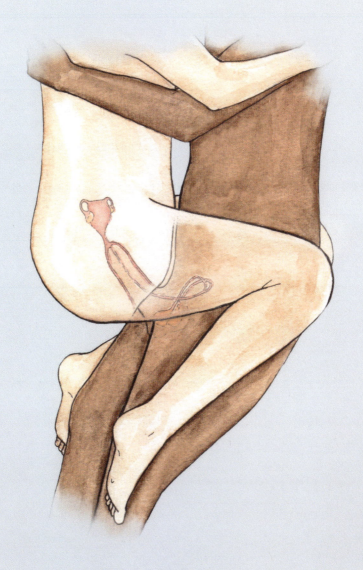

HOW TO START A CONVERSATION ABOUT SEX

The hardest part of talking to kids about sex is getting started. It's normal to feel a little uncomfortable when you first start talking about sex with your child. We all do. Many of us didn't have comfortable conversations with our own parents, growing up. We don't have any helpful memories of what to do, just lots of memories of what not to do! Like with all new things, it will get easier. The more often you talk with your child about sex, the easier it will get.

2 WAYS TO START A DIFFICULT CONVERSATION

There are a couple of different approaches to getting started.

1. WAIT FOR THE RIGHT OPPORTUNITY.

You can familiarise yourself with the explanations about sex and then sit back and wait for the perfect opportunity to arise. This approach is perfect for subsequent conversations, but not for a first conversation about sex.

Why? Because the first conversation about sex is always the hardest one. Afterwards, you'll be surprised by how easy it actually was. And you'll notice that the more conversations you have about sex, the easier they get.

Think back to a difficult conversation that you've had in the past and how easy it was to keep putting it off, even when you had the perfect opportunity sitting right there in front of you!

So, instead of sitting around waiting for the 'perfect' time to talk about sex, it's up to you to get the conversation started.

2. START THE CONVERSATION.

The best approach with difficult conversations is to start them yourself.

It's ok if your first attempt is a little unpolished. Expect a few extra "um's" and long pauses. If your child is older, you might encounter some uncomfortable responses, but also be ready for some blank stares and indifference.

Some kids take a while to digest information, while some ask a million questions. Others may not seem phased at all.

The important thing is you've opened up the conversation. You've made the first step.

In the last year, I've had over a dozen conversations with my 9-year-old son about porn. The other day, as we sat waiting for the traffic lights to turn green, just opposite a local adultshop, my son asks me, 'What's P-O-R-N?'

My response was, 'PORN. Why?'

'That's what it says on the sign. So, what is it?' he asked.

I turned to him in disbelief. 'What, you don't know what porn is? We have talked about this before, you know.'

He looks at me solemnly and says 'Did we? So, what's porn?'

So, what's the point of this story? The point of the story is that our conversations don't have to be perfect! When kids hear information in a natural, everyday way, that is too much for them to absorb or understand; they'll simply become bored and turn their attention elsewhere. Which is what happened with my son whenever I talked to him about porn.

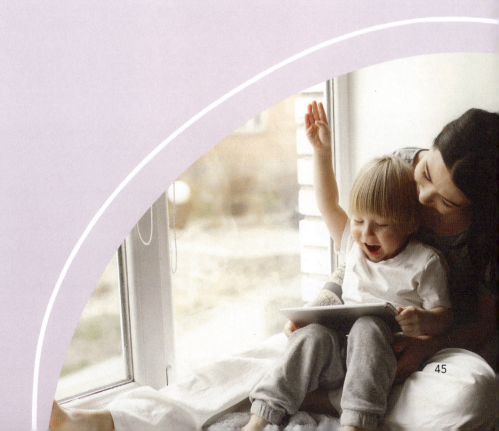

45

PLANNING THE CONVERSATION

Do your research. Familiarise yourself with the explanations about sex. Make sure there are no niggling little doubts about whether you are doing the right thing or not (or you'll never get started). Here are 13 of the most common reasons that parents don't talk to their kids about sex: https://sexedrescue.com/myths-and-facts-about-sex/

Make a plan. Identify why it's important that you talk to your child about sex. Then, write out all your thoughts, feelings and issues concerning the topic without censuring yourself. Decide what you want to tell your child about sex and how to start the conversation. Finally, think about the questions your child might ask and answer them on paper. Let your emotions flow freely during this planning period so that you can understand how you feel. Choose the main message that you wish to share.

Find out what your child already knows about sex. Ask your child, 'Do you know what sex is?' or, 'Have your friends talked about sex before?' This way, you'll know how much they already know. Which means you can gauge what else to tell them.

Check that they understood what you said. 'Does that make sense to you?'

Find out if they need more information. 'Do you have any questions?'

Be askable. Remind your child that they can talk to you about anything (no matter what). 'If you ever have any other questions or want to talk more about this, you can always ask me.'

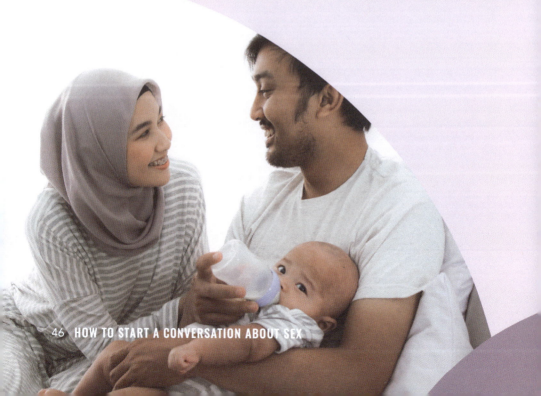

REMEMBERING WHAT TO SAY

Remembering what to tell your kids can be tricky. I still remember my first conversation with my kids about pornography. Porn was a conversation that I really didn't want to talk about, as it usually isn't nice sex. So, because I was stressing out so much about how the conversation would go, I wrote down on paper some dot points on what it was that I wanted to tell them. And it really did help!

This meant that I didn't have to worry about remembering what to say, and that instead I could focus on just saying it. And my kids didn't even notice that, at times, I was reading them something from a piece of paper.

So, do yourself a favour and write down the explanations that you plan to use. This way, you won't forget what to say!

TIPS:

- Grab some post-it notes and write one point per note. Attach them to the front of a book, then hold that in front of you when you talk to your child.

- Write the explanations you plan to use onto a piece of paper and stick them to your bathroom mirror or wall. Each night, as you stand there to brush your teeth, read them out to yourself so that they become familiar and a part of your vocabulary.

GETTING 'MORE COMFORTABLE'

Talking to kids about sex can make even the most confident parent feel uncomfortable.

It usually takes a little while to get used to talking about sex with your kids. You will be using words that you may not be used to saying, or talking about stuff that you may not normally talk to your kids (or anyone else) about.

The thing is, though, the more you talk, the easier it gets. Think of it like learning how to ride a bike. When you first get on, you feel quite unsure and clumsy. But the more you practice, the better you get at it. And before you know it, you are confident and riding like a professional!

Sex education is the same. We all feel awkward when we first start talking, but the more you talk, the sooner you start to feel more natural.

It is important to realize, though, that you will never be 100% comfortable with talking to your kids about sex. There will still be times when you feel uncomfortable, no matter how comfortable you think you are with talking about sex.

TIPS:

- Start by calling the gendered parts of the body their proper names, e.g., penis, testicles, scrotum, vulva, vagina, etc. You can find some suggestions on how to get started in this blogpost - https://sexedrescue.com/naming-private-parts/

- If you struggle with saying some of the words (like penis, vagina, sperm, sex), then practice saying the words aloud when by yourself. Pay attention to your reaction. Did you flinch or squirm when saying these words aloud? Repeat these words daily until you begin to feel more comfortable when saying them. Slowly start to use these words in your everyday conversations with your child.

- If you struggle with saying the explanations, then practice reading them aloud when by yourself. Pay attention to your reaction. Did you flinch or squirm when saying these words aloud? Practice saying the same explanations aloud a dozen or more times each, until you feel more comfortable saying them out loud. Then, try some different scripts and practice saying them aloud until you are comfortable with saying them. You could move onto saying them with a partner or a friend, and then your children.

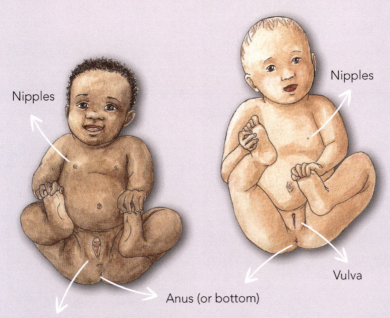

Nipples

Nipples

Vulva

Anus (or bottom)

This baby has genitals that look different to a penis or vulva.

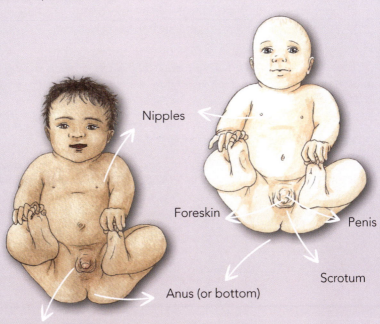

Nipples

Foreskin

Penis

Scrotum

Anus (or bottom)

Circumcised penis

DEALING WITH EMBARRASSMENT

It is common for both parents and kids to feel uncomfortable talking about sex. Luckily for you, it does get easier the more you do it. There are some things that you can do to help manage embarrassment.

TIPS:

- If you feel uncomfortable talking about sex, try saying, 'Some kids can feel really uncomfortable talking about sex with their parents. I totally get it! I feel awkward talking about it too. Maybe we can help each other get past the awkwardness.'

- If you feel embarrassed, try saying, 'I feel a bit uncomfortable talking about sex because my parents never talked with me about it. But this is an important subject, so I really want to talk with you about it.'

- If you are feeling self-conscious, avoid eye contact and start a conversation when you're in the car or doing the dishes.

- Try to keep your conversations simple and aim to share one piece of information with them. Decide what you want to talk about and think about the best way to casually bring up the topic.

- Take a deep breath and take your time to respond to questions. There is no rush! And if you don't know the answer, try saying something like, 'I don't know. So how about I find out and get back to you with answer?'

- Use humor. You don't have to make a joke about it, but laughing about sex shows that it is a normal topic.

- Get some books to read with your child. This way you don't have to stress about remembering what to say, as all the information is there in the book.

WHEN STARTING LATE

So, what's the best way to get started, when it feels like you may have left it too late?

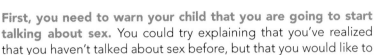

First, you need to warn your child that you are going to start talking about sex. You could try explaining that you've realized that you haven't talked about sex before, but that you would like to change that.

- I've realised lately that you're growing up really fast and that we haven't talked about sex. Since we haven't talked about it before, I'd like to start.

- I've been reading a book about sex education. I know we haven't talked about sex before, but I'm going to try to change that, so we can have conversations about it.

Second, explain why you haven't talked to them about sex before.

- Sex is something that my parents didn't talk about very much when I was a kid.

- I've always worried that I would get it all wrong or do as bad a job as my parents did.

- I've always been worried about saying too much or too little, or even saying the wrong thing.

- Talking about sex makes me feel really uncomfortable.

Third, explain what is going to change.

- I want us to be able to talk about anything. So, you are going to hear me talking about sex. If you have any questions or want to talk about something, I want you to know that I am always available.

IDEAS FOR TALKING ABOUT SEX

There are a few different ways to talk about sex with your child. Try to pick just one to start with, rather than trying to do them all. Choose one that feels comfortable, or like something you may already be doing. For example, if you already buy books for your child to read together, then buying a children's book about sex is a great way to start.

USE A BOOK

Books make explaining sex a lot easier, mainly because they contain the facts that you don't need to remember. Plus, the information in books is usually accurate, reliable, and written age-appropriately in language that your child will understand.

If you have yet to read a book about sex with your child, there are a few tricks that make it easier. The most important thing to remember is to make sure you first look at it by yourself. This blogpost - https://sexedrescue.com/reading-sex-education-books/ - will provide you with more tips.

You can find my recommendations for books here:

- Children's books that talk about how babies are made (without any mention of sexual intercourse) - https://sexedrescue.com/age-appropriate-books-about-where-babies-come-from/

- Children's books that talk about sexual intercourse - https://sexedrescue.com/childrens-books-about-how-babies-are-made/

- Children's books that talk about sex in an inclusive way - https://sexedrescue.com/inclusive-sex-education-books/

- Children's books that talk about all the other topics pertaining to sex education - https://sexedrescue.com/sex-education-books-for-children/

- Age-by-age list of sex education books - https://sexedrescue.com/sex-education-books-for-children/#ages

CONVERSATION STARTERS

I found this book at the library today that talks about how babies are made. Let's read it together.

This is a book that talks about sex. Did you want to have a look at it, and then we'll read it together tonight?

I heard about a book on the radio that talks about sex. So, I bought a copy for us to read together.

I have a special book for us to read tonight. It is about where babies come from.

Your Aunt Mary leant me a book that your cousins loved to read when they were your age. Let's sit down and read it.

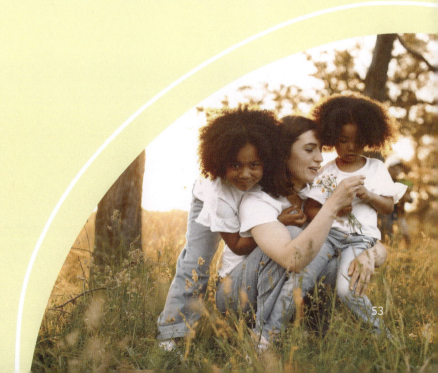

53

TEACHABLE MOMENTS

An easy way to talk to your child about sex is to find an everyday situation and turn it into an opportunity to teach something. At first you might find teachable moments a little bit hard to find, so you can learn more about Teachable Moments on my website, where I share many examples - https://sexedrescue.com/everyday-examples-of-spontaneous-teachable-moments/

TIPS:

* Write yourself a reminder and post it in a highly visible spot in the house or even on the steering wheel in the car. I do this when I want to talk about a particular topic (e.g., sexting) so that I remember to keep my eyes and ears open for the perfect opportunity to start talking about it.

When getting started, try to think of one topic that you would like to talk about, such as where babies come from. Then start looking for everyday opportunities to chat about babies. It could be some baby ducks at the local park, a new puppy, a pregnant person, or a baby doll. Once you start looking, you will find opportunities for talking, and teachable moments, everywhere.

CONVERSATION STARTERS

Look at those baby ducks over there. They are with their mother. How do you think she made them? Did she make them by herself? Or did she need some help?

Look at this magazine. It has a story about your favourite singer. He is gay, but he has a new baby. How do you think that happened?

Did you hear the words of that song just then? Do you know what they were talking about? They were talking about sex.

I heard a story on the radio today about how important it is for kids to understand how babies are made. How do you think babies are made?

Did you like the new puppy that your friend's dog had? Can you remember the last time we saw her dog, and she had a big fat tummy? Well, those puppies grew inside the mother dog's uterus. How do you think those puppies got inside the mother dog?

Did you hear that rude word just then, that that person just shouted out? They said the 'F-word,' (or fuck). Do you know what that word means?

Can I have a look at your baby doll? Have you ever wondered how babies are made?

Look at that lady with the big belly. She is pregnant. Do you know what that means?

OPENING LINES

Here are some opening lines that may help with starting a conversation about sex with your child. Don't forget that you probably already have a standard 'opener' that you are already using for awkward conversations. Mine is, 'Hey mate, …'

Remember when you asked me about…

Have you heard any of your friends talking about sex?

Let's learn about a new word and what it means. The word is 'sex.'

I realised that we haven't really talked yet about how babies are made.

Remember when we were talking about…

Have you ever wondered how you were made?

I found this book today. Let's read it together.

Do you know what sex is?

CONCLUSION

This book has provided you with a starting point. It has told you what to say to your child about sex and how to say it.

But it has also given you something else that is even more important - and priceless.

This book has given you the opportunity to strengthen your relationship with your child.

What I have found is that once parents start talking with their kids about sex, that they also start talking with them about other tricky topics like love and relationships.

Yes, you are still sharing facts with your child. Which means their decisions will be based on accurate information (instead of ignorance). But your conversations are strengthening your relationship with your child.

And because you are talking to your child about sex, they are growing up knowing you're a parent they can turn to with their questions, worries, concerns and problems.

And that is what makes these conversations priceless!

So, before you go, I want you to remember this…

It is okay to feel awkward. And the more you talk, the less awkward you'll begin to feel.

Start off simple. Start with language that is familiar, and as you feel more comfortable, slowly start to expand your vocabulary and become more inclusive.

It is many conversations. This isn't a 'one and done' conversation! You'll be having many conversations that you'll keep on repeating.

You don't have to be perfect. It's okay to forget things and to even say the wrong things. The benefit of having many conversations is that you can add in or correct yourself the next time!

Short conversations are just as effective as long ones. Don't feel as if all your conversations about sex have to be deep and meaningful. They don't. What matters is that you're having open and honest conversations about sex.

Use a book. Seriously, if you're worried about forgetting what to say or that you'll get it wrong, then start off by reading a book. Life is meant to be easy…not hard! And guess what? My first conversation with my own kids about sex started with a book!

The conversation is more important than the facts. When your child is an adult, they won't remember all the facts that you shared with them. What they'll remember is that they had a parent whom they could talk to about anything!

So, start talking!

Cath

RESOURCES

To find **more tools to help you** with sex education, you can go to: https://sexedrescue.com/products/

To find a comprehensive list of **sex education books for your child** to read, you can go to: https://sexedrescue.com/sex-education-books-for-children/

To ask questions about sex education and to connect with other parents on the same journey, you can **join my free parent Facebook group:** https://www.facebook.com/groups/thatparentgroup/

To receive regular information about sex education, you can sign up for my **parent newsletter**: https://sexedrescue.com/newsletter/

Plus, you will find **videos, articles and lots more** at Sex Ed Rescue: https://sexedrescue.com

REFERENCES

An Overview of Child Development Theories by Angela Oswalt. Mental Health Services of Southern Carolina. Accessed 7 August 2018 https://www.mhsso.org/poc/view_doc.php?type=doc&id=7918&cn=28

Child Sexual Development by Loretta Haroian. Electronic Journal of Human Sexuality, Volume 3. Accessed 6 October 2017 http://www.ejhs.org/volume3/Haroian/body.htm

Handbook of Child and Adolescent Sexuality: Developmental and Forensic Psychology. Edited by Daniel S. Bromberg and William T. O'Donohue. 2013. Elsevier. Academic Press. Oxford.

How to Talk to Kids about Babies, Birth, and Puberty: Tips to foster conversations from toddler to teen by Crystal de Freitas. 2012. eFrog Press.

Information by Age. Alberta Health Services. Accessed 7 August 2018. https://teachingsexualhealth.ca/parents/information-by-age/

Is This Normal? Understanding Your Child's Sexual Behaviors by Holly Brennan and Judy Graham. 2012. Family Planning Queensland: Fortitude Valley.

Sexual Development in Childhood edited by John Bancroft. 2003. Indiana University Press: Bloomington.

Understanding Your Child's Sexual Behaviour: What's Natural and Healthy by Toni Cavanagh Johnson. 1999. New Harbinger Publications, Inc. Oakland

Where do I start? Supporting healthy sexual development in early childhood by Family Planning Queensland. 2009. Family Planning Queensland: Fortitude Valley.

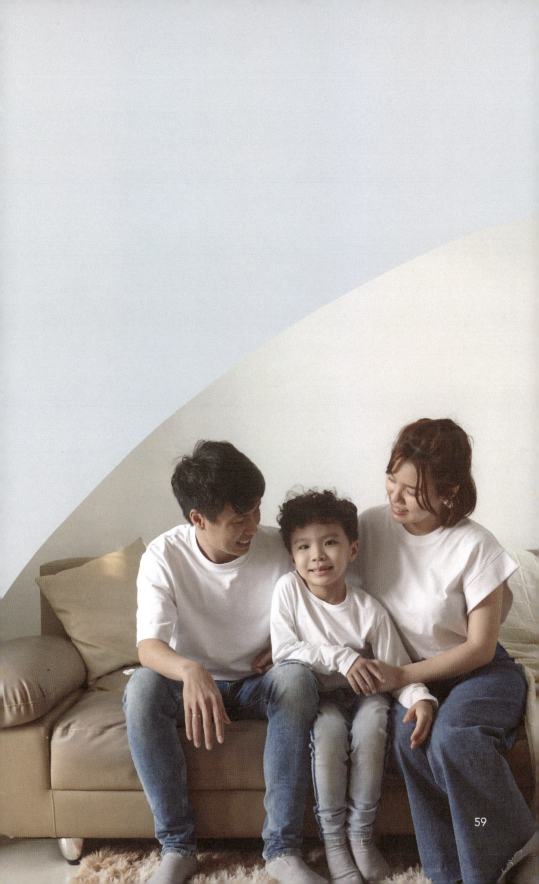

APPENDIX: AN ILLUSTRATED GUIDE
COMMON EXPLANATIONS
Uses language that many of us are familiar with

WHERE DO BABIES COME FROM?

**THIS PERSON LOOKS LIKE THEY HAVE
A BIG STOMACH BUT THEY DON'T.**

THEY HAVE A BABY GROWING INSIDE THEIR UTERUS.

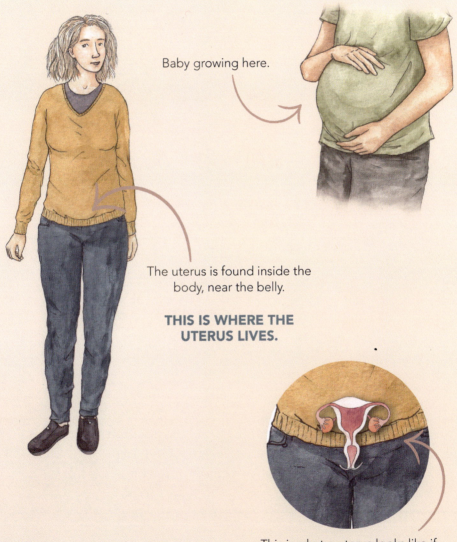

Baby growing here.

The uterus is found inside the
body, near the belly.

**THIS IS WHERE THE
UTERUS LIVES.**

This is what a uterus looks like if
you could see inside the body.

WHAT MAKES A BABY?

YOU NEED THREE THINGS TO MAKE A BABY.

Sperm, an egg, and a place for the baby to grow (the uterus).

This is what a sperm looks like up close.

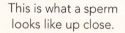

This is what an egg looks like up close.

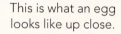

This is what the uterus looks like inside the body.

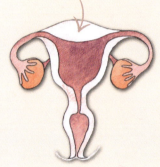

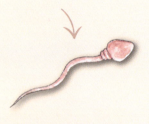

Another name for the egg is ovum.

Another name for the uterus is womb.

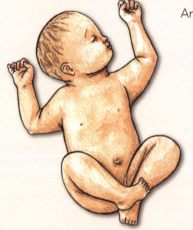

A BABY WILL START TO GROW WHEN THE SPERM JOINS WITH AN EGG.

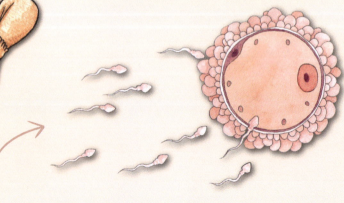

A sperm has joined with an egg.

WHERE DO THE SPERM & EGG COME FROM?

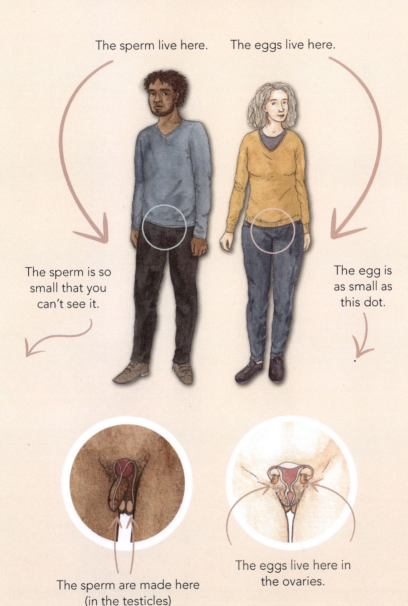

The sperm live here.

The eggs live here.

The sperm is so small that you can't see it.

The egg is as small as this dot.

The sperm are made here (in the testicles)

The eggs live here in the ovaries.

HOW DO THE SPERM & EGG MEET?

THERE ARE LOTS OF WAYS TO MAKE A BABY.

The sperm will travel from the testicles through the penis and into the vagina.
They use their wriggly tails to swim inside, where they might meet the egg.

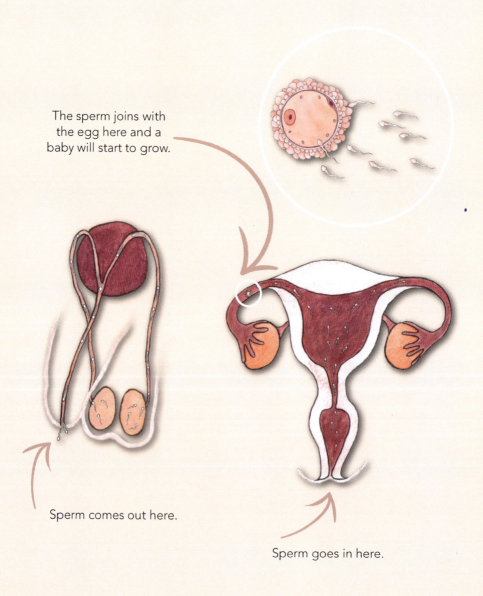

The sperm joins with
the egg here and a
baby will start to grow.

Sperm comes out here.

Sperm goes in here.

WHAT IS SEXUAL INTERCOURSE?

A man and a woman can make a baby by having sexual intercourse (or sex).

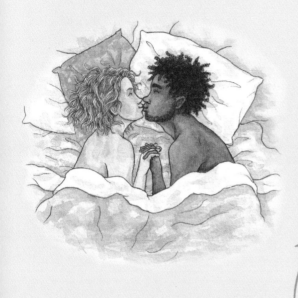

They will kiss and cuddle until the penis becomes hard and pokes out.

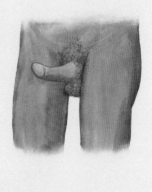

This is called an erection. An erection happens when the penis becomes hard and pokes out.

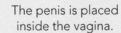

The penis is placed inside the vagina.

The sperm then travels from the testicles through the penis and into the vagina. The sperm swims into the uterus and fallopian tubes, where they might meet an egg.

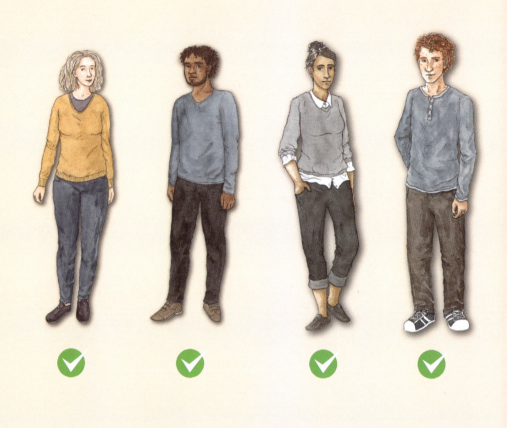

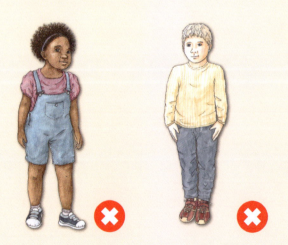

Sex is only for adults—not children!

WHAT ARE THE NAMES OF THE DIFFERENT BODY PARTS?

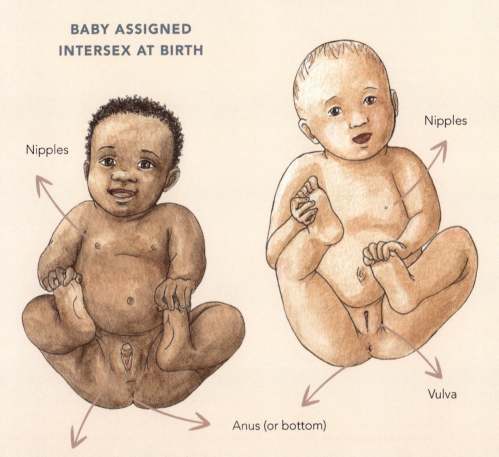

BABY ASSIGNED FEMALE AT BIRTH

BABY ASSIGNED INTERSEX AT BIRTH

Nipples

Nipples

Vulva

Anus (or bottom)

This baby has genitals that look different to a penis or vulva.

Sometimes a baby is born with genitals that look different. They might look different on the outside and/or inside of their body. When this happens, the baby is usually assigned intersex at birth.

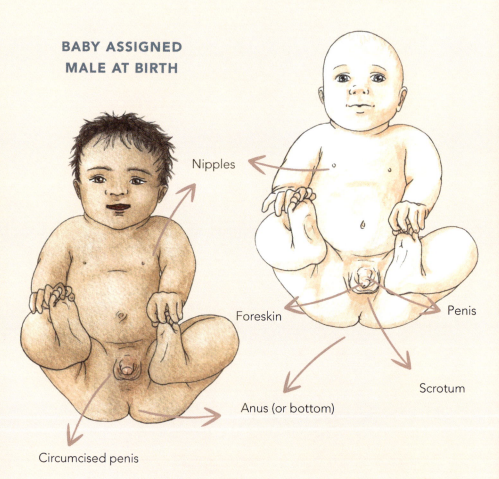

BABY ASSIGNED MALE AT BIRTH

BABY ASSIGNED MALE AT BIRTH

Nipples

Foreskin

Penis

Anus (or bottom)

Scrotum

Circumcised penis

Some penises look different because they have the foreskin removed. This is called circumcision and it is done for religious or medical reasons. It might happen when they are a baby, a child or an adult.

INCLUSIVE EXPLANATIONS

Uses language that is inclusive for trans gender and nonbinary people

WHERE DO BABIES COME FROM?

**THIS PERSON LOOKS LIKE THEY HAVE
A BIG STOMACH BUT THEY DON'T.**

THEY HAVE A BABY GROWING INSIDE THEIR UTERUS.

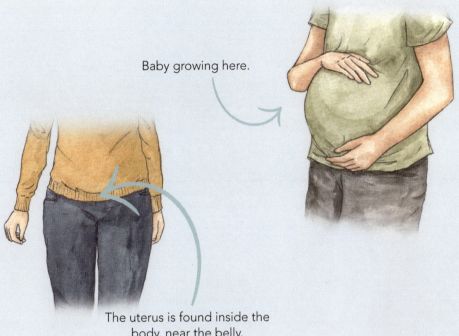

Baby growing here.

The uterus is found inside the
body, near the belly.

**THIS IS WHERE THE
UTERUS LIVES.**

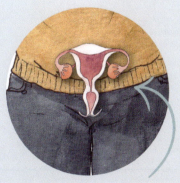

This is what a uterus looks like if
you could see inside the body.

WHAT MAKES A BABY?

YOU NEED THREE THINGS TO MAKE A BABY.

Sperm, an egg, and a place for the baby to grow (the uterus).

This is what a sperm looks like up close.

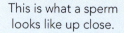

This is what an egg looks like up close.

This is what the uterus looks like inside the body.

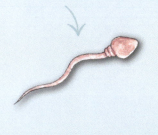

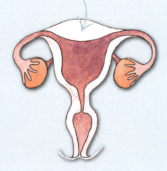

Another name for the egg is ovum.

Another name for the uterus is womb.

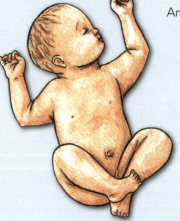

A BABY WILL START TO GROW WHEN THE SPERM JOINS WITH AN EGG.

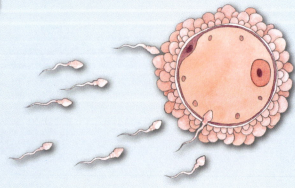

A sperm has joined with an egg.

WHERE DO THE SPERM & EGG COME FROM?

The sperm live here.

The eggs live here.

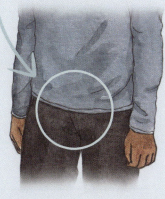

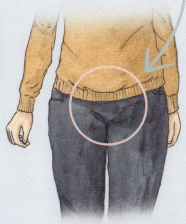

The sperm is so small that you can't see it.

The egg is as small as this dot.

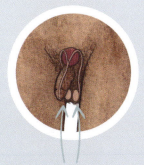

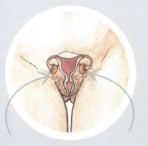

The sperm are made here (in the testicles)

The eggs live here in the ovaries.

HOW DO THE SPERM & EGG MEET?

THERE ARE LOTS OF WAYS TO MAKE A BABY.

The sperm will travel from the testicles through the penis and into the vagina.
They use their wriggly tails to swim inside, where they might meet the egg.

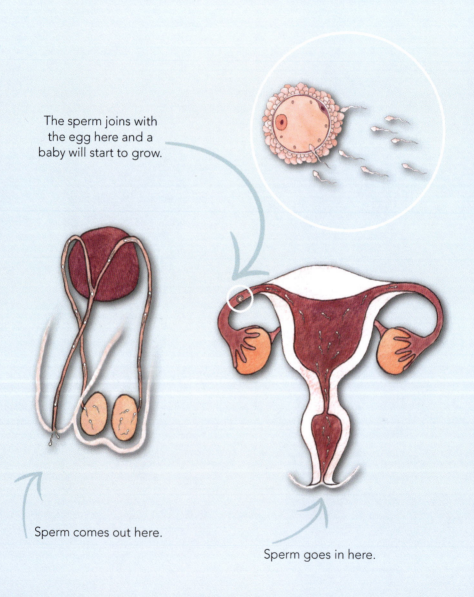

The sperm joins with
the egg here and a
baby will start to grow.

Sperm comes out here.

Sperm goes in here.

Sometimes, the sperm or egg might not work properly, or a person might not have an egg or sperm of their own. Alternatively, a person might be unable to grow a baby inside their body.

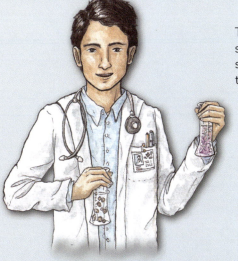

To get around these problems, someone might give them an egg or sperm, or offer to grow a baby inside their own uterus for them.

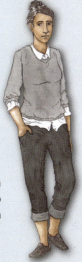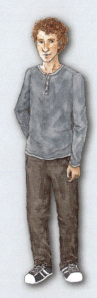

A doctor can help by placing the sperm inside the uterus. They may need to help the sperm and egg join together (this can happen inside or outside the body!).

Pictured are some of the special equipment doctors might use when helping people make a baby.

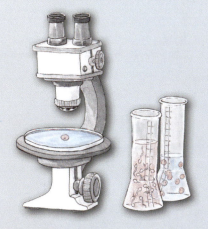

Some people might need special medicine to help them make a baby.

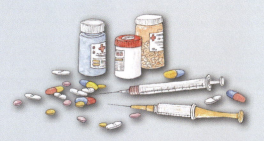

WHAT IS SEXUAL INTERCOURSE?

A person with a vagina and a person with
a penis can make a baby by having sex.

They will kiss and cuddle
until the penis becomes
hard and pokes out.

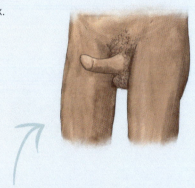

This is called an erection. An erection happens
when the penis becomes hard and pokes out.

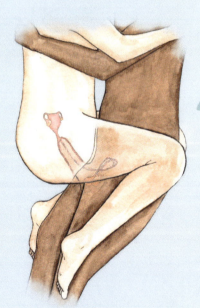

The penis is placed
inside the vagina.

The sperm then travels from the testicles through
the penis and into the vagina. The sperm swims
into the uterus and fallopian tubes, where they
might meet an egg.

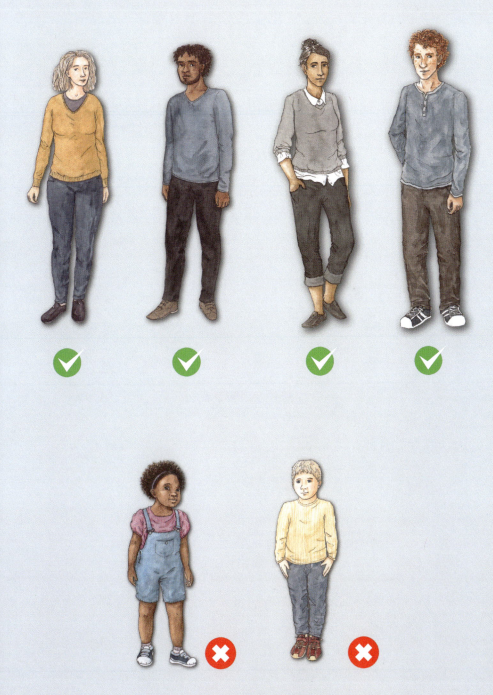

Sex is only for adults—not children!

WHAT ARE THE NAMES OF THE DIFFERENT BODY PARTS?

BABY ASSIGNED FEMALE AT BIRTH

BABY ASSIGNED INTERSEX AT BIRTH

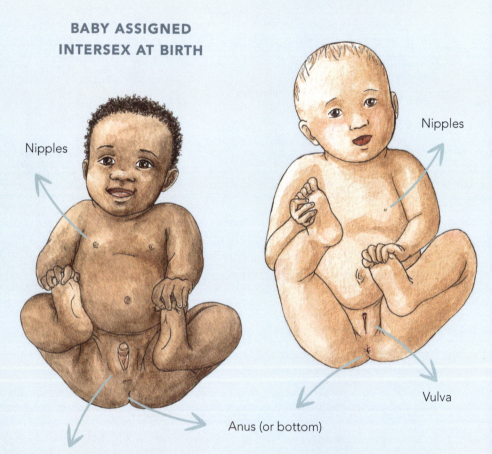

Nipples

Nipples

Vulva

Anus (or bottom)

This baby has genitals that look different to a penis or vulva.

Sometimes a baby is born with genitals that look different. They might look different on the outside and/or inside of their body. When this happens, the baby is usually assigned intersex at birth.

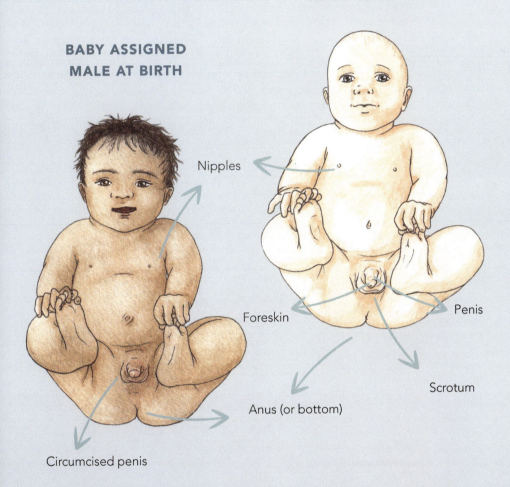

BABY ASSIGNED
MALE AT BIRTH

BABY ASSIGNED
MALE AT BIRTH

Nipples

Foreskin

Penis

Scrotum

Anus (or bottom)

Circumcised penis

Some penises look different because they have the foreskin removed. This is called circumcision and it is done for religious or medical reasons. It might happen when they are a baby, a child or an adult.

ABOUT CATH HAKANSON

Cath Hakanson has been talking to clients about sex for the past 25 years as a nurse, midwife, sex therapist, researcher, blogger and educator. She's spent the past 15 years trying to unravel why parents (herself included) struggle with sex education. Her solution was to create Sex Ed Rescue, an online resource that simplifies sex education and helps parent to empower their children with the right information about sex, so kids can talk to their parents about anything, no matter what.

Cath has lived all over Australia but currently lives in Perth with her partner, 2 children, and ever-growing menagerie of pets. Despite having an unusual profession, she bakes, sews, and knits for sanity, collects sexual trivia, and tries really hard not to embarrass her children in public. Well, most of the time anyway!

To find out more about Sex Ed Rescue, go to https://sexedrescue.com

MORE RESOURCES FROM SEX ED RESCUE THAT WILL HELP YOU TO HAVE SHAME-FREE CONVERSATIONS WITH YOUR CHILD ABOUT LOVE, SEX, RELATIONSHIPS AND GROWING UP!

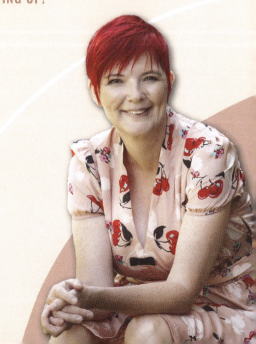

Printed in Great Britain
by Amazon

85526837R00047